DEFEATING DIABETES

EMPOWER YOUR HEALTH,
REVERSE TYPE 2, PREDIABETES
AND SHATTER MYTHS.

By

DR. ELVIRA S. GRAVES

TABLE OF CONTENTS

Disclaimer

Introduction

In the quiet of the night, when the world slows down and the day's hustle fades away, a moment of reflection often visits those living with diabetes. In this silence, the reality of the condition whispers it's truths—truths of challenge, resilience, and hope. This book is born from those whispered truths and the shared experiences of millions who navigate the complexities of diabetes every day.

A Personal Journey Through Diabetes

Meet Maya. At 53, she was a vibrant artist, a loving mother, and an active community member. Diabetes wasn't part of her plan. Yet, it crept in silently, manifesting through fatigue she attributed to her busy life. It wasn't until a routine check-up that she faced the unexpected diagnosis: Type 2 diabetes. Maya's story isn't unique; it mirrors the journey of many who find their lives intertwined with this condition. But it's Maya's response that turns her story into a beacon of encouragement. She took charge, educated herself, altered her diet, embraced exercise, and found strength she didn't know she had. Today, Maya's diabetes is well-managed, and she's more energetic than ever—her paintings are more vibrant with life.

The Purpose and Importance of This Book **"Defeating Diabetes: Empower Your Health, Reverse Type 2, Prediabetes, and Shatter Myths"** is more than just a title; it's a mission statement. This book aims to be your ally in understanding diabetes, a guide through the fog of misinformation, and a testament to the power of informed choices. It's crafted to empower you, the reader, with knowledge, to inspire success stories, and to equip you with practical tools for managing or even reversing diabetes.

An Overview of Diabetes

Diabetes is a global health concern with far-reaching impacts. It's a condition where the body either doesn't produce enough insulin or can't use it effectively, leading to elevated levels of glucose in the blood. There are three main types:
- **Type 1 Diabetes**: An autoimmune condition where the body attacks its insulin-producing cells.
- **Type 2 Diabetes**: The most common form, often associated with lifestyle factors and genetics.
- **Gestational Diabetes**: Occurs during pregnancy and usually resolves after birth.

The statistics are sobering. Over 422 million people worldwide live with diabetes, and it's the seventh leading cause of death globally. Yet, amidst these numbers lie misconceptions that cloud public understanding—myths that diabetes is always a result of poor lifestyle choices or that it's a life sentence of restriction and decline.

This book aims to shatter those myths. It's a journey into the heart of diabetes, guided by science, personal stories, and a steadfast belief in the potential for change. Together, we'll explore the realities, confront the challenges, and celebrate the victories. Because when it comes to diabetes, knowledge isn't just power—it's empowerment.

Welcome to "Defeating Diabetes." Your journey to empowerment starts here.

Chapter 1: Figuring Out Diabetes

Diabetes is an ongoing condition that influences millions around the world. It happens when the body can't use or produce insulin as expected, prompting raised degrees of glucose in the blood. Understanding diabetes is urgent for overseeing and possibly turning around its belongings.

What is Diabetes?

At its center, diabetes is about the body's battle with insulin, a chemical created by the pancreas. Insulin assists cells with retaining glucose from the blood to use as energy or store for some time. At the point when this framework flounders, it prompts diabetes. Diabetes is a constant (enduring) ailment that influences how your body transforms food into energy. Your body separates most of the food you eat into sugar (glucose) and delivers it into your circulation system. At the point when your glucose goes up, it flags your pancreas to deliver insulin. Insulin behaves like a key to allow the blood to sugar into your body's cells for use as energy. With diabetes, your body doesn't make sufficient insulin or can't use it as well as it should. At the point when there isn't sufficient insulin or cells quit answering insulin, an excessive amount of glucose stays in your circulatory system. After some time, that can cause serious medical issues, like coronary illness, vision misfortune, and kidney infection.

Kinds of Diabetes

There are three essential kinds of diabetes, each with unmistakable causes and executive techniques:

Type 1 Diabetes: An immune system condition where the body's insusceptible framework goes after the insulin-delivering cells' response and prevents your body from making insulin. Roughly 5-10% of individuals who have diabetes have type 1. Type 1 diabetes can be analyzed at whatever stage in life, and side effects frequently proliferate. Assuming that you have type 1 diabetes, you'll have to take insulin consistently to make due. At present, nobody knows how to forestall type 1 diabetes. in the pancreas. Individuals with type 1 diabetes require everyday insulin infusions to make due.

Type 2 Diabetes: The most well-known structure, where the body doesn't utilize insulin appropriately, prompting insulin obstruction. Over the long run, the pancreas can't make sufficient insulin to keep blood glucose at typical levels. Type 2 diabetes can frequently be dealt with through lifestyle changes and medicine. With type 2 diabetes, your body doesn't utilize insulin well and can't keep glucose at typical levels. Around 90-95% of individuals with diabetes have type 2. It was created over numerous years and is typically analyzed in

grown-ups (yet an ever-increasing number of kids, adolescents, and youthful grown-ups). You may not see any side effects, so it's critical to get your glucose tried assuming you're in danger. Type 2 diabetes can be forestalled or postponed with a sound way of life changes, for example, Getting in shape, Eating quality food, and Being dynamic.

Gestational Diabetes: This type happens during pregnancy and for the most part settles after birth. Nonetheless, it builds the gamble of creating type 2 diabetes further down the road. On the off chance that you have gestational diabetes, your child could be at a higher gamble for medical issues. Gestational diabetes generally disappears after your child is conceived. In any case, it builds your gamble for type 2 diabetes sometime down the road. Your child is bound to have corpulence as a youngster or high schooler and foster sort 2 diabetes further down the road.

The Science Behind Glucose, Insulin, and the Body's Energy The board The Science Behind: Insulin Opposition Insulin is a chemical that guides in the guideline of your body's glucose levels and digestion (the cycle through which food is changed over into energy). Insulin is delivered by your pancreas and delivered into your blood. It permits your body to consume sugar for energy and afterward store the rest. Insulin opposition happens when cells in your muscles, fat, and liver neglect to answer insulin and can't use glucose from your blood for energy. To redress, your pancreas creates additional insulin and your glucose levels ascend over the long run. Insulin obstruction can prompt issues like diabetes, elevated cholesterol, and hypertension. "You can't see that you have insulin obstruction by how you feel. You'll have to get a blood test that checks your glucose levels."

There are likewise three fundamental kinds of insulin. Effective insulin is immediately

consumed into the circulatory system from fat underneath your skin and is utilized to oversee glucose levels during feasts and snacks as well as to treat high blood glucose. Middle-of-the-road-acting insulin is retained all the more leisurely and has a more extended term of activity. It is utilized to control glucose levels for the time being, during fasting, in the middle between eating. Long-acting insulin is gradually ingested, has a low pinnacle influence, and has a supported level impact that endures most of the day. It's likewise used to keep glucose levels stable for the time being, during fasting, in the middle between feasts. Little endeavors, like eating better food varieties and expanding active work, can assist with switching insulin obstruction and forestall or delay type 2 diabetes in patients with prediabetes.

The body's energy the executives rotate around glucose, a straightforward sugar obtained from the food we eat. Insulin assumes an urgent part in permitting glucose to enter cells. At the point

when insulin capability is debilitated, glucose stays in the circulatory system, prompting high glucose levels. After some time, this can harm different organs and frameworks.

Risk Variables and Side Effects of Prediabetes and Type 2 Diabetes

Prediabetes is a condition where glucose levels are higher than ordinary but not yet sufficiently high to be analyzed as diabetes. It's an admonition sign, showing a high gamble of creating type 2 diabetes. Risk factors incorporate weight, dormancy, family ancestry, and age. Side effects might incorporate expanded thirst, continuous pee, weakness, and obscured vision.

Ebb and Flow Exploration on Diabetes

Research keeps on propelling comprehension we might interpret diabetes. Late investigations have distinguished new hereditary markers and are investigating novel medicines focused on the basic reasons for diabetes. These headways hold

a guarantee for better administration and likely remedies for diabetes later on. ADA-subsidized specialists utilize the cash from their honors to direct basic diabetes research. In time, they distribute their discoveries to advise individual researchers regarding their outcomes, which guarantees that others will expand upon their work. At last, this cycle drives advances to forestall diabetes and to help individuals troubled by it. In 2018 alone, ADA-supported researchers distributed more than 200 articles connected with their honors.

Identification of another Player with type 1 Diabetes risk

Type 1 diabetes is brought about by an immune system assault of insulin-delivering beta-cells. While hereditary qualities and the climate are known to assume significant parts, the hidden variables making sense of why the insusceptible framework erroneously perceives beta-cells as unfamiliar isn't known.

Now, Dr. Delong has found an expected clarification. He found that proteins called Crossbreed Insulin Peptides (HIPs) are tracked down in beta-cells of individuals with type 1 diabetes and are perceived as unfamiliar by their safe cells. Indeed, even after diabetes begins, resistant cells are as yet present in the blood that assault these HIPs.

Then, Dr. Delong needs to decide whether HIPs can act as a biomarker or potentially even be designated to forestall or treat type 1 diabetes. Pastry specialist, R. L., Rihanek, M., Hohenstein, A. C., Nakayama, M., Michels, A., Gottlieb, P. A., Haskins, K., and Delong, T. (2019). Hybrid Insulin Peptides Are Autoantigens in Type 1 Diabetes. Diabetes, 68(9), 1830-1840.

Deciding the job of BPA in type 2 diabetes risk Numerous manufactured synthetics have penetrated our food framework during the period in which places of diabetes have flooded. Information has recommended that one specific

manufactured synthetic, bisphenol A (BPA), might be related to an expanded gamble of creating type 2 diabetes. In any case, no concentrate to date has decided if utilization of BPA changes the movement of type 2 diabetes in people. Results revealed for the current year by Dr. Hagobian showed that for sure when BPA is regulated to people in a controlled way, there is a quick, direct impact on glucose and insulin levels.

Now, Dr. Hagobian needs to lead a bigger clinical preliminary including openness to BPA over a more extended period to decide exactly what BPA means for glucose and insulin. Such outcomes are critical to guarantee the expulsion of synthetic substances adding to persistent illnesses, including diabetes.

Hagobian, T. A., Bird, A., Stanelle, S., Williams, D., Schaffner, A., and Phelan, S. (2019). Pilot Concentrate on the Impact of Orally Regulated Bisphenol A on Glucose and Insulin Reaction in

Nonobese Grown-ups. Diary of the Endocrine Society, 3(3), 643-654.

Understanding the science of body-weight guidelines in kids

Deciding the organic instruments controlling body weight is significant for forestalling type 2 diabetes. The ascent in youth stoutness has made this much more critical. Social examinations have shown that reactions to food utilization are changed in kids with stoutness, however, the basic natural components are obscure. This year, Dr. Schur tried changes in mind and hormonal reactions to dinner in typical weight and stout youngsters. Results from her review show that hormonal reactions in stout youngsters are typical following a feast, however, reactions inside the cerebrum are decreased. The absence of reaction inside the cerebrum might incline them toward overconsumption of food or trouble with weight reduction.

With this data within reach, Dr. Schur needs to examine how this data can be utilized to treat corpulence in youngsters and lessen diabetes.

Roth, C. L., Melhorn, S. J., Elfers, C. T., Scholz, K., De Leon, M. R. B., Rowland, M., Kearns, S., Aylward, E., Grabowski, T. J., Saelens, B. E., and Schur, E. A. (2019). Focal Sensory system and Fringe Chemical Reactions to a Dinner in Youngsters. The Diary of Clinical Endocrinology and Digestion, 104(5), 1471-1483.

Chapter 2: The Fantasies And Bits of Insight About Diabetes

Diabetes is covered in a horde of fantasies that can darken reality and upset the successful administration of the condition. Understanding these legends and the real factors behind them is urgent for anybody moved by diabetes.

Normal Fantasies and Their Truths
Fantasy: Eating sugar causes diabetes.
Truth: While inordinate sugar admission can prompt weight gain, which is a gamble factor for type 2 diabetes, sugar alone doesn't cause diabetes. The improvement of diabetes is

impacted by a blend of hereditary and way-of-life factors.

fantasy: Diabetes is not a serious infection.
Truth: Diabetes is a critical worldwide medical problem that can prompt serious inconveniences on the off chance that are not overseen as expected, including coronary illness, stroke, kidney disappointment, and vision misfortune.

Fantasy: Individuals with diabetes can't eat desserts or chocolate.
Truth: Individuals with diabetes can eat desserts and chocolate if they are represented inside their general dinner plan and sugar intake[3].

fantasy: You can get diabetes from another person.
Truth: Diabetes isn't infectious. It can't be contracted like a cold or influenza.

The Reality of Diabetes

The executives and Inversion Compelling diabetes the board spins around an extensive methodology that incorporates way-of-life changes, medicine adherence, and customary observing of blood glucose levels. A few stages for overseeing and possibly switching diabetes include:

-Executing Part Control: Overseeing segment sizes can assist with controlling calorie consumption and keeping a solid weight.

- Expanding Fiber Admission: Fiber dials back carb processing and sugar retention, helping with glucose control.

-Taking on a Decent Eating routine: An eating routine low in handled food varieties and high in natural products, vegetables, and entire grains upholds by and large well-being.

- Ordinary Actual work: Exercise assists the body with utilizing insulin all the more proficiently and can bring down blood glucose levels.

-Stress Decrease: Ongoing pressure can influence glucose levels, so overseeing pressure is a significant part of diabetes care.

-Quality Rest: Satisfactory rest is fundamental for general well-being and can assist with directing glucose levels.

Experiences from Clinical Exploration and Well-qualified Sentiments Late clinical exploration has taken critical steps in grasping diabetes among executives. Studies have shown the significance of patient schooling, well-being proficiency, and the job of medical services suppliers in supporting patients with diabetes. Specialists underline the requirement for individualized care plans, recognizing the one-of-a-kind difficulties every individual with diabetes faces. They additionally feature the significance of open, deferential correspondence and social skills in diabetes care.

Way of Life Changes as an Answer:
A few specialists contend that with a huge way of life changes, especially in diet, type 2 diabetes can be switched. Neil Barsky, who switched his own kind 2 diabetes, stresses the significance of understanding the job of diet and nourishment in overseeing glucose levels. The

Job of Diet: A veggie-lover diet has been proposed by certain specialists as a way to forestall, treat, and, surprisingly, invert type 2 diabetes. Research demonstrates that veggie lovers might diminish their gamble of diabetes by 78% compared with the people who consume meat every day.

Clinical Point of view: As per clinical experts, type 2 diabetes is reversible under specific circumstances, particularly when an individual embraces the sound way of life changes. Only prescriptions are sufficient not to invert it, and without a solid way of life changes, the condition will advance.

Never Past Time to Begin: Specialists additionally say that beginning rolling out certain improvements is rarely past the point of no return. While prior mediation can prompt improved results, upgrades in glucose control and general well-being can be accomplished at any phase of the sickness. It's tied in with finding the right methodology and making economical ways of life changes.

These conclusions feature the agreement that while type 2 diabetes is a serious medical issue, it can frequently be overseen and possibly switched through the devoted way of life changes, especially those connected with diet and exercise. It's critical to talk with medical services suppliers to make a customized plan for overseeing diabetes.

All in all, scattering fantasies and embracing insights about diabetes can engage people to assume command over their well-being. With

the right information and backing, living great
with diabetes is an attainable objective.

Chapter 3: Nourishment And Diabetes

The Effect of an Ill-advised Diet on Diabetes
An ill-advised diet is a main supporter of the turn of events and compounding of diabetes. Eats less carbs high in refined sugars, unfortunate fats, and handled food varieties can prompt weight gain, irritation, and insulin obstruction, which are all chance elements for type 2 diabetes. Eating unnecessary measures of unfortunate food varieties has been distinguished as a huge driver of the worldwide flood in type 2 diabetes than the absence of healthy food varieties.

The job of Diet in Overseeing and Switching Diabetes

Diet assumes a basic part in overseeing and possibly switching diabetes. A reasonable eating routine that incorporates different supplements can assist with controlling glucose levels, further develop insulin responsiveness, and decrease the gamble of inconveniences. Research has demonstrated the way that dietary changes can prompt preferable A1c results over some normal diabetes medications[7]. A plant-based diet, specifically, is powerful in controlling glucose and may try to reverse diabetes.

Many individuals inquire as to whether I might at any point switch my diabetes with diet. From an indicative viewpoint, when you have type 2 diabetes you have it. Yet, from a physiological stance, many individuals can and do invert their diabetes, regardless of how long they've had diabetes. 'Diabetes reduction' and 'diabetes inversion/turned around' are two ordinarily exchangeable terms utilized in logical examination. Being 'all around controlled' is one more term that is much of the time utilized by dietitians and specialists. Even though it is comparative, being 'very much controlled' can have a somewhat unique significance to having diabetes that is 'disappearing' or 'switched.' For example, 'reduction' and 'switched' would most regularly show that an individual has accomplished and is keeping up with typical blood glucose and is off all/most meds, accomplishing these results dominatingly through diet and way-of-life changes.

Being very much controlled may show that an individual uses a mix of diet, way of life, and different diabetes drugs as a method for accomplishing better blood glucose levels. The job of diet What we cannot deny is that how you eat assumes a basic part in assisting with the "inversion" of diabetes. Dietary change alone can prompt preferred A1c results over recommending normal prescriptions like Metformin. Dietary change diminishes the gamble of diabetes complexities and further develops other well-being biomarkers, for

for example, weight, circulatory strain, and cholesterol. In recent years, research has shown that 2 dietary strategies have come with the best results:

Dietary Rules for Prediabetes and Type 2 Diabetes Dietary treatment is a major part of diabetes care. It includes individualized directing to improve glycemic control, accomplish weight-the-board objectives, and further develop cardiovascular gamble factors. The American Diabetes Affiliation suggests an eating routine that incorporates different supplements and thick food varieties, for example, non-starchy vegetables, entire grains, lean proteins, and solid fats, while restricting added sugars and refined grains.

Feast Arranging and Recipes for a Diabetes-Accommodating Eating Routine Feast-making arrangements for a diabetes-accommodating eating regimen ought to zero in on entire food sources and incorporate more non-starchy vegetables like broccoli, spinach, and green beans. It's likewise essential to incorporate less added sugars and refined grains. For instance, a feast plan could begin with a plate filled half with non-starchy vegetables, one quarter with lean protein, and one quarter with entire grains or dull vegetables.

Recipes for a Diabetes-Accommodating Eating Routine

Numerous scrumptious recipes fit into a diabetes-accommodating eating routine. A few models include Chicken Veggie Bundles: A straightforward and sound mix of herbed chicken and vegetables prepared in foil parcels. Darkened Tilapia with Zucchini Noodles: A light and tasty dish that matches zesty fish with low-carb zucchini noodles. Turkey Cabbage Stew: A good and nutritious stew loaded up with ground turkey, cabbage, carrots, and tomatoes.

Concluding, sustenance assumes a fundamental part in the administration and possible inversion of diabetes. By complying with wholesome rules and integrating quality feast arranging and recipes into day-to-day existence, people with diabetes can move toward working on their well-being and prosperity.

Chapter 4: Exercise And Way Of Life Changes

The Effect of Active Work on Glucose Levels
 Active work is a vital part of overseeing diabetes. The practice affects glucose control. During active work, muscles use glucose for energy, which brings down glucose levels. Normal activity likewise increments insulin responsiveness, meaning the body's phones can utilize accessible insulin all the more productively to ingest glucose during and after movement. This can bring down glucose levels for as long as 24 hours or more after exercising.

Exercise Suggestions for People with Diabetes

The American Diabetes Affiliation suggests somewhere around 150 minutes of moderate-force high-impact action each week.

This can be fanned out north of a few days, without any than two back-to-back days without exercise to keep up with consistent glucose levels[2]. Moderate-power exercises could incorporate energetic strolling, cycling, swimming, or group activities. It's vital to begin gradually, particularly if new to work out and step by step increment the span and power.

There are a couple of ways that exercise brings down blood glucose (otherwise called glucose): Insulin awareness is expanded, so your muscle cells are better ready to utilize any suitable insulin to take up glucose during and after action. At the point when your muscles contract during movement, your phones can take up glucose and use it for energy regardless of whether insulin is accessible. This is how exercise can assist with bringing down blood glucose for the time being. What's more, when you are dynamic consistently, it can likewise bring down your A1C.

Grasping Your Blood Glucose and Exercise
The impact actual work has on your blood glucose will shift contingent on how long you are dynamic and numerous different variables. Actual work can bring down your blood glucose as long as 24 hours or more after your exercise by making your body more sensitive to insulin. Get comfortable with how your blood glucose answers work out. Checking your blood glucose level all the more frequently when exercising can assist you with seeing the advantages of movement. You additionally can utilize the aftereffects of your blood glucose verifies how your body responds to various exercises. Understanding these examples can assist you with keeping your blood glucose from going excessively high or excessively low.

Hypoglycemia and Actual Work

Individuals taking insulin or insulin secretagogues (oral diabetes pills that make your pancreas make more insulin) are in danger of hypoglycemia if insulin protein or carb

admission isn't changed with work out. Looking at your blood glucose before doing any actual work is essential to forestall hypoglycemia (low blood glucose). Converse with your diabetes care group (specialist, attendant, dietitian, or drug specialist) to see whether you are in danger of hypoglycemia. Assuming that you experience hypoglycemia during or after working out, treat it right away: Adhere to the 15-15 guidelines:

1. look at your blood glucose.
2. Assuming your perusing is 100 mg/dL or lower, have 15-20 grams of sugar to raise your blood glucose. This might be
4 glucose tablets (4 grams for every tablet),
1 glucose gel tube (15 grams for each gel tube),
4 ounces (1/2 cup) of juice or normal pop (not diet), or
1 tablespoon of sugar or honey

3. Take a look at your blood glucose again following 15 minutes. Assuming that it is still under 100 mg/dL, have one more serving of 15 grams of starch.

4. Rehash these means like clockwork until your blood glucose is somewhere around 100 mg/dL. If you have any desire to proceed with your exercise, you will typically have to enjoy some time off to treat your low blood glucose. Check to get back in the saddle up over 100 mg/dl before beginning to practice once more. Remember that low blood glucose can happen during or long after actual work. It is bound to happen if you:

- Take insulin or an insulin secretagogue
- Skip meals
- Exercise for quite a while
- Exercise arduously

Assuming hypoglycemia obstructs your workout daily practice, converse with your medical services supplier about the best therapy plan for you. Your supplier might recommend eating a little nibble before you exercise or they might make an acclimation to your medication(s). For individuals participating in

lengthy-term workouts, a blend of these two routine changes might be important to forestall hypoglycemia during and after workouts.

 Work-out Schedules for People with Diabetes A balanced work-out daily schedule for people with diabetes could include;

High-impact Exercise: Exercises like strolling, swimming, or moving for no less than 30 minutes as a general rule.

Opposition Preparing: Utilizing loads or obstruction groups no less than two times per week to further develop muscle strength.

 Adaptability and Equilibrium: Yoga or extending practices improve adaptability and equilibrium, which is especially significant for more seasoned grown-ups.

Way of Life Alterations to Help Diabetes

The executive's Way of life changes are pivotal for overseeing diabetes successfully. These include

 -**Smart dieting:** A decent eating routine, wealthy in supplements, low in fat, and moderate in calories.

-**Ordinary Check-Ups**: Observing glucose levels and counseling medical services suppliers consistently.

-**Stress The board**: Procedures like reflection or advising to oversee pressure. Sufficient Rest: Guaranteeing 7-9 hours of value rest every evening. Smoking End: Staying away from tobacco use, which can increment glucose levels and lead to intricacies.

Finally, integrating normal active work into one's day-to-day practice, alongside another way of life changes, can essentially further develop glucose control and generally speaking

well-being in people with diabetes. It's a strong step towards a better existence with diabetes.

Chapter 5: Clinical Administration Of Diabetes

Drugs and Their Components of Activity
The administration of diabetes frequently includes various drugs, each managing various systems to control glucose levels. Compelling diabetes the executives requires a comprehensive methodology that tends to the actual parts of the condition as well as the profound and mental difficulties that might emerge. It's critical to work intimately with medical care suppliers to foster an administration plan that is practical and compelling for long-haul wellbeing.

Biguanides (e.g., Metformin): Diminish how much glucose is created by the liver. Sulfonylureas (e.g., Glimepiride, Glipizide): Animate the pancreas to deliver more insulin. Meglitinides (e.g., Repaglinide, Nateglinide): Increment insulin creation in the pancreas in a glucose-subordinate way. Thiazolidinediones (e.g., Pioglitazone): Further develop insulin responsiveness in muscle and fat cells and decrease glucose creation in the liver. DPP-4 Inhibitors (e.g., Sitagliptin, Saxagliptin): Slow the inactivation of incretin chemicals, which increments insulin delivery and diminishes glucagon levels. SGLT2 Inhibitors: Block glucose reabsorption in the kidneys, prompting glucose to be discharged in the pee.

Checking Glucose Levels and Involving Innovation in Diabetes Care

Checking glucose levels is significant for overseeing diabetes. There are a few techniques and innovations accessible:

Blood Glucose Meters: Convenient gadgets that action glucose levels in a little drop of blood, normally taken from the fingertip. Constant **Glucose Screens (CGMs)**: Gadgets that give continuous glucose readings, taking into account more thorough glucose pattern checking.

Innovation in diabetes care has progressed essentially, with apparatuses like robotized insulin conveyance frameworks and diabetes self-administration applications that assist patients with better dealing with their condition. Diabetes innovation is the term used to portray the equipment, gadgets, and programming that individuals with diabetes use to help with self-administration, going from way-of-life changes to glucose checking and treatment changes. By and large, diabetes innovation has been separated into two principal classes: insulin managed by needle, pen, or siphon (likewise called persistent subcutaneous insulin imbuement), and glucose as surveyed by blood glucose observing (BGM) or nonstop glucose checking (CGM). Diabetes innovation has extended to incorporate robotized insulin conveyance (Help) frameworks, where CGM-informed calculations balance insulin conveyance, as well as diabetes self-administration support programming filling in as clinical gadgets. Diabetes innovation, when combined with instruction, follow-up, and support, can work on the lives and soundness of individuals with diabetes; in any case, the intricacy and quick development of the diabetes innovation scene can likewise be a boundary to execution for the two individuals with diabetes and the medical care group.

General Gadget Standards (Recommendations)

1. The type(s) and choice of gadgets ought to be individualized given an individual's particular requirements, inclinations, and expertise level. In the setting of a person whose diabetes is somewhat or entirely overseen by another person

(e.g., a small kid or an individual with mental hindrance or finesse, psychosocial, or potentially actual constraints), the guardian's abilities and inclinations are necessary to the dynamic cycle.

2. While recommending a gadget, guarantee that individuals with diabetes/guardians get starting and continuous schooling and preparation, either face to face or from a distance, and progressing assessment of method, results, and their capacity to use information, including transferring/sharing information (if relevant), to screen and change treatment.

3. Individuals with diabetes who have been utilizing ceaseless glucose checking, consistent subcutaneous insulin mixture, and additionally robotized insulin conveyance for diabetes the executives ought to have proceeded with access across outsider payers, paying little mind to progress in years or A1C levels.

4. Understudies ought to be upheld at school in the utilization of diabetes innovation, for example, consistent glucose observing

frameworks, ceaseless subcutaneous insulin implantation, associated insulin pens, and computerized insulin conveyance frameworks, as endorsed by their medical care group.

5. Commencement of persistent glucose observing, ceaseless subcutaneous insulin imbuement, as well as mechanized insulin conveyance right off the bat in the treatment of diabetes can be gainful relying upon an individual's/parental figure's requirements and inclinations.

Blood Glucose Checking (Recommendations)

1. Individuals with diabetes ought to be given blood glucose observing gadgets as shown by their conditions, inclinations, and treatment. Individuals utilizing nonstop glucose observing

gadgets should likewise approach blood glucose checking consistently.

2. Individuals who are on insulin utilizing blood glucose observing ought to be urged to check their blood glucose levels when proper in light of their insulin treatment. This might incorporate checking while fasting, before dinners and bites, after feasts, at sleep time, before working out, when hypoglycemia is thought, in the wake of treating low blood glucose levels until they are normoglycemic when hyperglycemia is thought, and previously and keeping in mind that performing basic errands like driving.

3. Medical services experts ought to know about the distinctions in exactness among blood glucose meters — just meters endorsed by the U.S. Food and Medication Organization (or similar administrative offices for other topographical areas) with demonstrated exactness ought to be utilized, with unexpired

strips bought from a drug store or authorized wholesaler.

4. Even though blood glucose checking in people on non insulin treatments has not in every case shown clinically critical decreases in A1C, it very well might be useful while changing sustenance plans, actual work, or potential prescriptions (especially drugs that can cause hypoglycemia) related to a treatment change program.

5. Medical services experts ought to know about drugs and different elements, like high-portion L-ascorbic acid and hypoxemia, that can slow down glucose meter exactness and give clinical administration as shown.

<u>When to Think about Insulin Treatment</u>
<u>Insulin treatment is thought about when</u>:

Blood glucose levels can't be controlled with diet, workouts, and different prescriptions. The patient has type 1 diabetes or high-level sort 2 diabetes. The HbA1c level is higher than 10% at finding, or blood glucose levels are reliably high.

In conclusion, the clinical administration of diabetes includes a blend of drugs, ordinary observing of glucose levels, and the utilization of cutting-edge innovation to guarantee ideal control of the condition. Insulin treatment is a basic part for some, especially when different medicines are lacking. Patients need to work intimately with their medical care suppliers to decide the best administration procedure for their singular necessities.

Chapter 6: Conquering Difficulties and Remaining Persuaded

Living with diabetes presents a novel arrangement of difficulties that can influence actual well-being, yet close to home prosperity as well. This part investigates how to explore these difficulties with strength and keep up with inspiration for viable diabetes management.

Adapting to the Profound Parts of Diabetes (emotional)

Diabetes can be a close-to-home rollercoaster, with sentiments going from forswearing and outrage to pressure and sorrow. Perceiving these feelings as a characteristic piece of living with an ongoing condition is significant. Here are a few systems to adapt:

-**Recognize Your Sentiments**: Allow yourself to strongly feel and express your feelings.
-**Look for Proficient Assistance**: Consider conversing with a guide or clinician who can give procedures to oversee pressure and profound well-being.
-**Practice Care**: Methods like contemplation can assist you with remaining present and lessen uneasiness.
-**Put forth Reasonable Objectives**: Separate your administration plan into reachable advances. -**Observe Little Triumphs**: Recognize each achievement, regardless of how little.
- **Track down Your Why**: Remember the individual motivations behind why dealing with your diabetes means a lot to you.

Diabetes doesn't simply influence you truly, it can influence you genuinely as well. Whether you've recently been determined or you've lived to have diabetes for quite a while, you might require support for every one of the feelings you're feeling. This could be pressure, feeling low and discouraged, or copied out. Individuals around you can feel all of this as well. Anything you're feeling, you are in good company. Here is some data you could view as accommodating - you could jump at the chance to impart it to your loved ones as well.

CENTER AROUND THINGS YOU HAVE SOME CONTROL OVER

Assuming you're thinking of yourself as stressed, it could assist with attempting to zero in on the things that you have some control over in your life. Here are a few hints:
-Realize your SICK day rules
 -go to arrangements when your medical services group asks you to
- look at your work approaches around ailment and downtime
- keep significant numbers convenient

-know the side effects of COVID and what to do assuming you start to feel sick ----Ensure you have supplies and repeat prescriptions up to date
-Care for your body attempt to settle on quality food decisions, be dynamic, get sufficient rest, and clean up more
-regularly lookout for Recipe Locater for groundbreaking
-thoughts try to care for your psyche assuming that you're remaining at homestay in contact with loved ones if possible
-express no to things you don't want to and request help on your day off
-get your report from solid sources but at the appropriate time.

THINGS YOU HAVE NO CONTROL OVER

- Zeroing in your brain on things beyond your control won't change things. This can prompt concern, so tenderly attempt to divert your consideration.

- You may be feeling anxious because your condition might make you more helpless against becoming unwell. Be that as it may, you don't have command over this, so attempt to be thoughtful and merciful to yourself on the off chance that you are unwell.

- On the off chance that you are sick, you might need to miss work, school, or arrangements. This is OK and the best thing to do is to care for yourself as well as other people.

- You could likewise be agonizing over some diabetes arrangements being dropped or finding it hard to get hold of your medical care group. There may be elective choices, similar to telephone or video arrangements, so investigate these. Most arrangements aren't dire, however on the off chance that your diabetes group requires to see you they will reach out for

an arrangement. You should attempt to go to these.

- Not having the option to get what you need from the shops can be distressing. You have no control over the accessibility of provisions. Attempt to be patient and make an effort not to overreact to purchase. Assuming you are experiencing issues getting food supplies, we are making a valiant effort to help you. Figure out the thing we're doing.

- It's difficult to stop sensations of nervousness and stress, and these are typical reactions given the ongoing conditions. You have zero control over your sentiments, yet you have some control over how you manage them. Discussing how you're feeling could help.

The emotional well-being noble cause Brain has assembled some helpful data

about dealing with your emotional well-being during this time as well.

DISCUSSING HOW YOU FEEL

Discussing diabetes and how it's affecting you isn't simple 100% of the time. It tends to be difficult to get everything rolling or find somebody you want to open up to. Perhaps you don't feel like you really want to discuss anything or you would rather not trouble anybody. In any case, offloading some of what you're feeling has countless advantages both for yourself and those near you.

Systems for Keeping up with Inspiration and Adherence to Treatment Plans

Remaining spurred can be intense, particularly when the monotonous routine of diabetes the executives feels overpowering. To stay focused:
- **Building an Emotionally supportive network:** Family, Companions, and Medical Services

Experts A solid emotionally supportive network is essential for overseeing diabetes. It can give profound solace, down-to-earth help, and important data.
- **Loved ones**: Teach them about diabetes so they can offer the right help. - Medical care Group: Fabricate a relationship with your PCPs, medical caretakers, and dietitians who grasp your necessities.
- **Support Gatherings**: Associate with other people who are going through comparative encounters.

Lastly, beating the profound and persuasive difficulties of diabetes requires a diverse methodology. By recognizing feelings, laying out feasible objectives, and building major areas

of strength for an organization, you can keep an uplifting perspective and remain roused in your excursion with diabetes. Keep in mind that you're in good company, and with the right systems and backing, you can deal with your diabetes.

Chapter 7: Win Over Diabetes - Examples Of Overcoming Adversity And Motivational Excursions

In this part, we dive into the cheering accounts of people who have dealt with diabetes directly and arisen triumphantly. Through their meetings and individual accounts, we uncover the procedures and attitudes that have empowered them to oversee or try and oppose their condition. These stories act as encouraging signs and are loaded with useful guidance for those leaving on a comparative excursion.

The Excursion of Emma:

A Story of Industriousness Emma was determined to have type 2 diabetes at 42 years old. At first, wrecked, she chose to assume command over her well-being. She began by rolling out little improvements, for example, consolidating a day-to-day walk and lessening sweet bites. After some time, these progressions became propensities, and Emma saw a critical improvement in her glucose levels. Her story is a demonstration of the force of gradual change.

Mark's Marathon Journey: A Step-by-Step Chronicle

The Diagnosis That Started It All

Mark's life took an unexpected turn when he was diagnosed with type 1 diabetes. The news came as a shock, but it also ignited a spark within him to take charge of his health. He realized that he had to make significant lifestyle changes if he wanted to manage his condition effectively.

The First Steps

Mark began by setting small, achievable goals. His first milestone was to walk 5,000 steps every day. As his fitness improved, he increased his target, and soon, walking turned into jogging. He kept a detailed log of his blood sugar levels to understand how exercise affected his condition.

Building Up Stamina

After a few months, Mark felt confident enough to join a local running club. Surrounded by fellow runners, he found both camaraderie and competition, which pushed him to go further. He participated in 5K runs, gradually moving up to 10Ks. With each race, his confidence soared.

The Marathon Decision

A year into his journey, Mark decided to set his sights on the ultimate challenge: running a marathon. He knew it would be tough, not just physically but also in managing his diabetes during the long hours of training and the race itself. He worked closely with his healthcare team to create a plan that would keep him safe.

Training Days

Mark's training regimen was rigorous. He ran five days a week, cross-trained, and rested adequately. Nutrition played a crucial role, and he learned to fuel his body correctly for endurance. He also mastered the art of adjusting his insulin doses on long-run days.

Race Day

The marathon day was a mix of nerves and excitement. Mark started strong, pacing himself and monitoring his glucose levels throughout. By the halfway point, he felt a surge of energy, knowing that every step was a victory over diabetes.

The Finish Line

Crossing the finish line was an emotional moment for Mark. It wasn't just about completing the marathon; it was about the journey that got him there. He proved to himself and others that diabetes could be managed and that it didn't have to stop anyone from achieving their dreams.

Post-Marathon Reflections
After the marathon, Mark became an advocate for diabetes awareness and fitness. He shared his story to inspire others, showing that with determination and the right support, anything is possible.

Lessons Learned
- **Education is Key**: Understanding the nature of diabetes is crucial. Knowledge empowers individuals to make informed decisions about their diet, exercise, and medication.
- **Support Systems Matter**: Having a network of friends, family, or a support group provides encouragement and accountability.
- **Consistency Over Perfection**: Consistent efforts in managing diabetes are more effective than

striving for perfection and feeling discouraged by setbacks.

Tips from the Pathways
- **Monitor Regularly**: Keep track of blood sugar levels to understand how different foods and activities affect your body.
- **Stay Active**: Find an activity you enjoy and make it part of your routine.
- **Healthy Eating**: Focus on a balanced diet with plenty of vegetables, whole grains, and lean proteins.

Conclusion

Charting the Course to Victory Over Diabetes
As we conclude "Defeating Diabetes: Empower Your Health, Reverse Type 2, Prediabetes, and Shatter Myths," we reflect on the empowering journey we've embarked upon together. This book has been a beacon of knowledge, debunking myths and illuminating the path to better health.

Key Takeaways
- **Diabetes is Not a Dead End**: We've learned that a diabetes diagnosis is not the end of the road but the beginning of a transformative journey.
- **Lifestyle is the Key**: The cornerstone of managing and reversing diabetes lies in lifestyle

modifications—balanced nutrition, regular exercise, and stress management.

- Knowledge is Power: Understanding the mechanisms of diabetes gives you the power to make informed choices about your health.

Empowerment for the Journey Ahead
You are equipped with the tools and understanding necessary to navigate the complexities of diabetes. Let this knowledge empower you to make choices that enhance your well-being and steer you toward a healthier future.

A Call to Action
Take the reins of your health. Implement the strategies outlined in this book, and remember that small steps can lead to significant changes. You have the potential to reverse type 2 diabetes and prediabetes, and it starts with the decision to act today.

Resources for Further Reading and Support

A curated selection of additional literature, online resources, and community support groups to continue your education and find encouragement.

"Defeating Diabetes" is more than a book; it's a companion on your journey to health. As you turn each page into action, remember that you are not alone. Together, we can shatter the myths and embrace a life of health and vitality.

IF YOU GOT VALUES FROM THIS BOOK, KINDLY DROP A POSITIVE REVIEW FOR ME. THANK YOU

ALSO CHECK SOME OF MY BOOK HERE..
https://www.amazon.com/author/elvygraves